THE
PRACTICAL GUIDE
TO DEMENTIA

Empowering Caregivers with Techniques to Support Cognitive Health, Foster Emotional Stability, and Minimize Stress in Dementia Care Settings

Juana H. Bennett

Copyright © 2024 Juana H. Bennett

All rights reserved.

No part of this publication may be reproduced, distributed, or transmitted in any form or by any means, including photocopying, recording, or other electronic or mechanical methods, without the prior written permission of the publisher, except in the case of brief quotations embodied in critical reviews and certain other noncommercial uses permitted by copyright law.

The Practical Guide to Dementia | **Juana H. Bennett**

Table of Contents

INTRODUCTION 6
CHAPTER 1: WHAT IS DEMENTIA? 10
   Definition and Overview 10
   Types of Dementia 12
      Alzheimer's Disease 12
      Vascular Dementia 14
      Lewy Body Dementia 15
      Frontotemporal Dementia 17
      Other Types 19
   Causes and Risk Factors 21
   Symptoms and Stages 23
CHAPTER 2: DIAGNOSIS AND ASSESSMENT ... 26
   Recognizing Early Signs 26
   Seeking Medical Help 28
   Diagnostic Tests and Tools 29
      Cognitive Assessments 29
      Imaging Tests 31
      Laboratory Tests 33
   Understanding the Diagnosis 35
   Communicating the Diagnosis to the Family 37
CHAPTER 3: TREATMENT AND MANAGEMENT 40
   Medical Treatments 40

Medications 40
Non-pharmacological Treatments 42
    Cognitive Stimulation Therapy (CST) 42
    Reminiscence Therapy 43
    Validation Therapy 45
    Music Therapy 46
    Physical Exercise 47
    Art Therapy 48
    Environmental Modifications 50
    Sensory Stimulation 51
    Social Engagement 52
Aromatherapy 53
Managing Co-existing Conditions 57

CHAPTER 4: DAILY LIVING AND CAREGIVING 60

Creating a Safe and Comfortable Environment 60
Daily Care Routines 61
    Personal Hygiene 62
    Dressing and Grooming 63
    Nutrition and Mealtime 63
    Daily Routine Caregiving Approach 64
Communication Strategies 65
Activities and Engagement 66
Managing Challenging Behaviors 66
    Aggression and Agitation 66

Wandering 67

Sleep Issues 68

CHAPTER 5: LEGAL AND FINANCIAL PLANNING 70

Understanding Legal Documents 70

Power of Attorney 70

Living Will 71

Guardianship 71

Financial Planning 72

Budgeting for Care 72

Insurance Options 73

Government Assistance Programs 74

CHAPTER 6: SUPPORT FOR CAREGIVERS 76

The Role of the Caregiver 76

Coping with Stress and Burnout 77

Finding Support Groups 78

Respite Care Options 78

Self-care for Caregivers 78

CHAPTER 7: RESOURCES AND SUPPORT 82

Professional Care Services 82

In-Home Care 82

Adult Day Care 82

Assisted Living and Nursing Homes 83

Community Resources 83

Local Support Organizations 83

National and International Organizations.............84

Online Resources and Tools.......................................85

CHAPTER 8: ADVANCES IN DEMENTIA RESEARCH 88

Current Research Trends 88

Breakthroughs in Treatment 90

Future Directions in Dementia Care.........................91

CHAPTER 9: PERSONAL STORIES AND CASE STUDIES 94

Real-life Experiences of Those Living with Dementia
....94

Caregiver Stories 95

Conclusion 98

Appendices..100

BONUS ALERT

Note that there's special bonus at the end of this guide. All you need to do is to scan the **QR Code** provided at the end of this book to access it.

INTRODUCTION

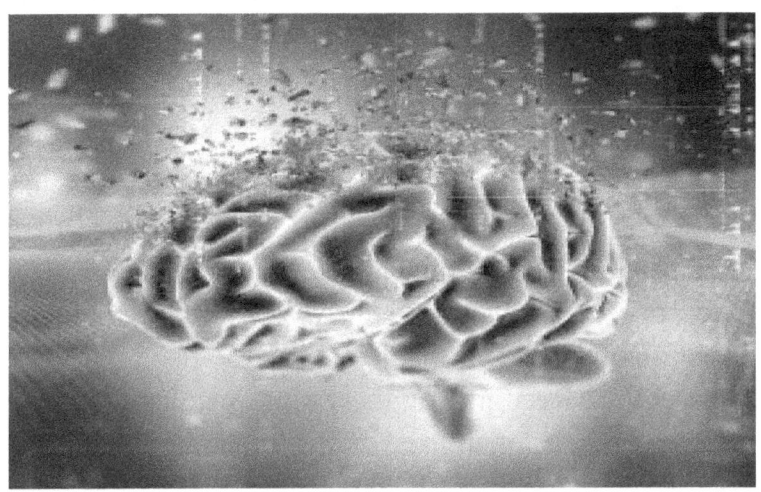

Dementia is a broad term that includes various cognitive impairments significantly disrupting everyday life and activities. It is not a singular ailment but rather a compilation of symptoms that might arise from several underlying conditions, such as Alzheimer's disease, vascular dementia, Lewy body dementia, and frontotemporal dementia. As the global population ages, the incidence of dementia is rising, making it a critical area of focus for healthcare professionals, caregivers, and families alike.

"The Practical Guide to Dementia" aims to provide comprehensive and accessible information to those affected by dementia, directly or indirectly. This guide addresses the diverse challenges of dementia, offering practical strategies for managing symptoms and improving quality of life. By covering a wide range of topics—from understanding the different types of dementia to navigating the complexities of daily care—this guide is an essential resource for caregivers, healthcare providers, and individuals with dementia.

One of the primary objectives of this guide is to demystify dementia and provide clear, actionable advice. It begins by explaining the medical and biological aspects of dementia, helping readers understand how and why cognitive decline occurs. The guide then delves into the early signs and symptoms, emphasizing the importance of early detection and intervention. Recognizing these signs can lead to more effective management and better outcomes for those affected.

Practical caregiving is at the heart of this guide. It offers detailed strategies for handling common behavioral and psychological symptoms of dementia, such as agitation, confusion, and memory loss. Tips on communication techniques, environmental modifications, and activities that promote cognitive engagement are included to help caregivers provide the best possible support. Additionally, the guide addresses caregiving's emotional and psychological impact, offering advice on self-care and stress management.

Legal and financial considerations are also covered, ensuring readers are well-informed about planning for the future. This includes information on setting up power of attorney, managing finances, and understanding the legal rights of individuals with dementia. By providing this crucial information, the guide aims to alleviate some of the burdens associated with the practical aspects of caregiving.

The Practical Guide to Dementia | **Juana H. Bennett**

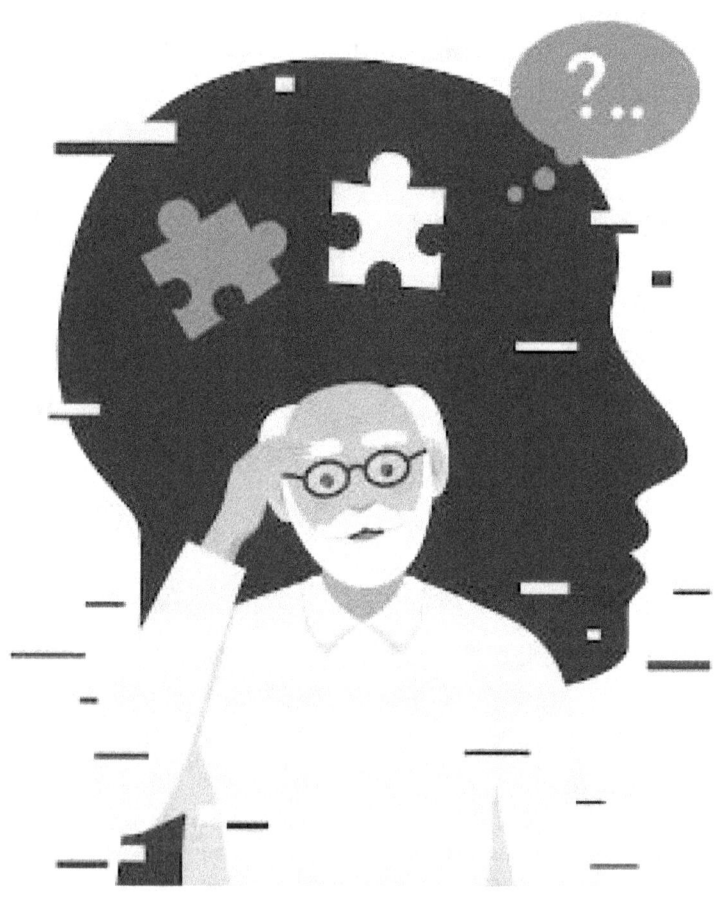

CHAPTER 1: WHAT IS DEMENTIA?

Definition and Overview

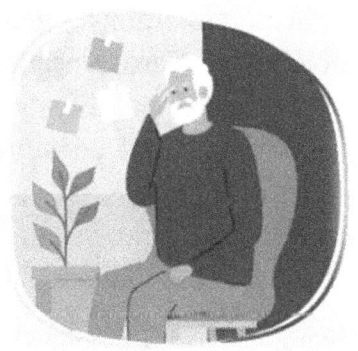

Dementia is a broad word used to describe various symptoms associated with cognitive decline, which interfere with daily functioning. It is a complex condition that encompasses several diseases. However, it is a syndrome characterized by deteriorating memory, thinking, behavior, and the ability to perform everyday activities. The most prevalent type of dementia is Alzheimer's disease, which accounts for 60-80% of cases. Other types include vascular dementia, Lewy body dementia, and frontotemporal dementia, each with distinct clinical features and underlying pathologies.

The onset of dementia is typically gradual, and the condition progresses over time. Early symptoms often include forgetfulness, difficulty finding words, losing track of time, and misplacing items. As dementia advances, individuals may experience severe memory loss, confusion, mood changes, difficulty communicating, and impaired judgment. Eventually, they may require full-time care and assistance with basic activities such as eating, dressing, and personal hygiene.

Dementia mainly affects older persons, although aging is not a natural aspect. As people age, their chance of having dementia rises, but it can also result from various medical conditions, genetic factors, and lifestyle choices. Cardiovascular diseases, diabetes, hypertension, and lifestyle factors such as smoking, excessive alcohol consumption, and lack of physical activity are known risk factors. Additionally, traumatic brain injuries and certain neurological conditions can promote the development of dementia.

Diagnosis of dementia involves a comprehensive medical assessment, including a detailed patient history, physical examination, neurological tests, cognitive and neuropsychological evaluations, and imaging studies such as MRI or CT scans. Early diagnosis is crucial for managing symptoms, slowing progression, and planning for the future. While there is currently no cure for dementia, treatments are available to alleviate symptoms and improve the quality of life for affected individuals. These include medications for cognitive symptoms and behavioral therapies to address mood and behavior changes.

The impact of dementia extends beyond the individual to families, caregivers, and society. Providing care for an individual with dementia may be physically, emotionally, and financially demanding. Support services, education, and resources for caregivers are essential components of dementia care. Furthermore, research into the prevention, treatment, and potential cure for dementia is ongoing, focusing on understanding the underlying mechanisms and developing effective interventions.

Types of Dementia
Alzheimer's Disease

Alzheimer's disease is a degenerative neurological ailment that typically affects older persons, progressively decreasing memory, cognitive function, and behavior. Named for Dr. Alois Alzheimer, who first recognized it in 1906, the illness is defined by developing two kinds of aberrant protein fragments in the brain: plaques of beta-amyloid protein outside neurons and tangles of tau protein within neurons. These buildups impede communication between brain cells, leading to their malfunction and ultimate death.

The symptoms of Alzheimer's disease often develop slowly and worsen over time, sometimes beginning with moderate forgetfulness and increasing to severe memory loss, disorientation, confusion about time and place, and changes in mood and behavior. As the condition proceeds, people may struggle with the duties of daily life and lose the capacity to identify loved ones.

Although the specific etiology of Alzheimer's disease is not entirely known, age is a significant risk factor. Other variables such as genetics, family history, and certain lifestyle factors, including cardiovascular health and education level, may also play a role. Current research reveals that a mix of genetic, environmental, and lifestyle variables contribute to the development of the condition.

Diagnosis of Alzheimer's disease needs a complete medical assessment, including medical history, cognitive tests, imaging scans (such as MRI or CT scans), and occasionally genetic testing to rule out other potential causes of symptoms. While there is no cure for Alzheimer's disease, medications are available to help control symptoms, slow down development, and enhance the quality of life for afflicted persons. These therapies often include drugs that temporarily improve cognitive function or regulate behavioral issues.

Caring for someone with Alzheimer's disease may be challenging and involves a multidisciplinary strategy combining healthcare experts, caregivers, and support networks. Care techniques frequently concentrate on establishing a secure and supportive environment, properly managing drugs, and providing emotional and practical assistance for the person and their caretakers.

Research into Alzheimer's disease continues to improve, with current research examining novel therapies, early detection techniques, and possibly prevention strategies. Public awareness and funding for research are crucial in tackling the rising impact of

Alzheimer's disease on individuals, families, and healthcare systems worldwide.

Vascular Dementia

Vascular dementia is a sort of dementia due to injury to the brain by limited blood flow. It is the second most prevalent kind of dementia after Alzheimer's disease. The brain needs a steady supply of oxygen and nutrients supplied by blood to operate correctly. When blood flow to the brain is diminished or obstructed, brain cells may be deprived of crucial nutrients and oxygen, leading to injury or death. This damage emerges as cognitive impairment and reductions in thinking ability.

The causes of vascular dementia frequently entail disorders that impact blood arteries throughout the body, including the brain. Conditions such as stroke, where an abrupt cessation of blood flow to the brain causes tissue damage, are a substantial risk factor. Tiny vessel disease, including damage to the small blood arteries deep inside the brain, may also contribute to vascular dementia. Other disorders that contribute to vascular dementia include high blood pressure, diabetes, high cholesterol, and heart disease, all of which may damage blood arteries and raise the risk of stroke or diminished blood supply to the brain.

Symptoms of vascular dementia may vary widely depending on the section of the brain affected and the extent of damage. Common symptoms include challenges with planning, organizing, and problem-solving, as well as slower thinking, issues with concentration, and memory deficits that are generally less severe than those in Alzheimer's disease. People with vascular dementia may also suffer mood swings, sadness, or changes in behavior.

Diagnosis of vascular dementia typically entails a complete medical history, neurological examination, and tests of cognitive function. Brain imaging methods such as MRI or CT scans may assist in detecting regions of damage or anomalies in the brain's blood vessels. Treatment focuses on reducing risk factors that lead to vascular injury, such as regulating blood pressure, managing cholesterol levels, and treating diabetes. Medications may also be recommended to control symptoms or avoid additional issues.

Managing vascular dementia frequently needs a multidisciplinary approach combining healthcare experts, therapists, and caregivers to address both the physiological and psychosocial components of the illness. Supportive techniques such as cognitive rehabilitation, occupational therapy, and emotional support for the person with dementia and their caregivers are vital in sustaining quality of life.

Lewy Body Dementia

Lewy body dementia (LBD) is a complicated and degenerative brain condition that impairs a person's ability to think, walk, sleep, and function independently. It is characterized by the formation of abnormal protein deposits termed Lewy bodies in the brain's nerve cells, which impede the brain's normal functioning. Named for Dr. Friedrich H. Lewy, who first found these aberrant protein deposits in the early 20th century, LBD is considered the second most frequent type of progressive dementia after Alzheimer's disease.

The symptoms of Lewy body dementia can vary widely among individuals but typically include cognitive impairment that fluctuates in severity, visual hallucinations, problems with movement and balance (resembling Parkinson's disease), sleep disturbances such as REM sleep behavior disorder (acting out dreams), and fluctuations in attention and alertness. These oscillations may frequently be more significant than those found in Alzheimer's disease when cognitive deterioration tends to advance more consistently.

Diagnosing Lewy body dementia may be problematic owing to its overlapping symptoms with other neurodegenerative conditions, including Alzheimer's disease and Parkinson's disease. A complete evaluation frequently comprises a detailed medical history, physical examination, neurological tests, and brain imaging scans to rule out other possible explanations.

Lewy body dementia does not have a treatment right now, and therapy focuses on controlling symptoms and enhancing quality of life. Medications may be provided to treat cognitive and movement problems; however, their efficacy might vary. Non-pharmacological therapies such as physical, occupational, and speech therapy may also assist in controlling symptoms and retaining independence for as long as feasible.

Caregiving for adults with Lewy body dementia may be challenging owing to the unexpected nature of symptoms and the requirement for specialized care. Caregivers frequently need information and help adequately handle the problems associated with the condition.

Research into Lewy body dementia is underway to understand its underlying causes better, create more reliable diagnostic methods, and investigate new therapies that might halt its development or ease symptoms. Clinical studies are vital for furthering understanding and improving treatment for those afflicted by this complicated and devastating illness.

Frontotemporal Dementia

Frontotemporal dementia (FTD) represents a spectrum of neurodegenerative illnesses defined by the progressive destruction of neurons in the frontal and temporal lobes of the brain. These areas affect personality, conduct, and language, making FTD unique from other kinds of dementia, like Alzheimer's disease. Typically hitting persons under the age of 65, FTD presents widely from person to person, causing difficulty in diagnosis and treatment.

The development of FTD is gradual, frequently beginning with minor changes in behavior, emotions, or linguistic skills. Early symptoms may include apathy, social retreat, disinhibition, or obsessive behaviors, indicating the damaged frontal lobe's involvement in controlling behavior and social conduct. In contrast, language variations of FTD might first appear with difficulties finding words, speech production problems, or grammatical mistakes owing to temporal lobe involvement.

As the illness advances, these symptoms worsen, impairing everyday functioning and interpersonal connections severely. Individuals with FTD may demonstrate substantial personality changes, lack of empathy, decreased judgment, and difficulties reading social signals. Language variations may grow into more severe aphasia, impairing verbal and receptive communication abilities.

The fundamental pathology of FTD includes aberrant protein accumulation inside brain cells, leading to their malfunction and ultimate death. These deposits frequently consist of tau protein (in instances known as tauopathies) or TDP-43 protein (in cases known as TDP-43 proteinopathies), producing particular patterns of neuronal death in afflicted brain areas.

Diagnosing FTD offers complications owing to its overlapping symptoms with other disorders and the range of presentations within the disorder itself. Neurological tests, cognitive evaluations, and imaging procedures like MRI or PET scans are critical for proper diagnosis, frequently demanding specialist review by neurologists or neuropsychiatrists.

Currently, no cure exists for FTD, and therapy focuses on managing symptoms and supporting afflicted persons and their families. This strategy incorporates a multidisciplinary team comprising neurologists, psychologists, speech therapists, and social workers to address cognitive decline, behavioral problems, and emotional well-being.

Other Types

Dementia comprises a variety of neurological illnesses beyond Frontotemporal, Alzheimer's disease, Vascular dementia, and Lewy body dementia. Each variety shows various symptoms and development patterns, adding to varied obstacles in diagnosis and therapy.

Parkinson's Disease Dementia (PDD): PDD is connected with Parkinson's disease (PD), a degenerative neurological illness affecting mobility. Over time, persons with PD may acquire cognitive decline, including memory loss, executive dysfunction, and difficulty with language. PDD often emerges in the latter stages of PD when motor symptoms become severe.

Huntington's Disease (HD): HD is a hereditary condition marked by abnormal movements (chorea), cognitive impairment, and mental symptoms. The cognitive symptoms of HD generally include decreased judgment, trouble with multitasking, and memory impairments. HD often presents in maturity, advancing over 10 to 25 years following the beginning.

Creutzfeldt-Jakob Disease (CJD): CJD belongs to prion disorders that cause rapid neurological degeneration. Symptoms include fast dementia, ataxia, muscular stiffness, and behavioral abnormalities. CJD advances swiftly, frequently resulting in mortality within a year after symptoms start.

Wernicke-Korsakoff Syndrome: This disorder is primarily caused by thiamine (vitamin B1) deficiency, frequently linked with prolonged alcohol usage or malnutrition. Wernicke's encephalopathy manifests with acute symptoms such as disorientation, ataxia, and ophthalmoplegia. If untreated, it may proceed to Korsakoff syndrome, characterized by severe memory loss, confabulation, and apathy.

Normal Pressure Hydrocephalus (NPH): NPH includes an abnormal accumulation of cerebrospinal fluid in the brain's ventricles, leading to cognitive impairment, urine incontinence, and gait abnormalities. Symptoms might match those of Alzheimer's or Parkinson's disease, making diagnosis problematic without imaging studies.

Mixed Dementia: Mixed dementia occurs when more than one kind of dementia is present concurrently, such as Alzheimer's disease and vascular dementia. This combination generally leads to more severe cognitive impairment and a quicker decline than any one kind of dementia alone.

Posterior Cortical Atrophy (PCA): PCA is an uncommon type of Alzheimer's disease where deterioration develops mainly in the brain's rear (posterior) parts, which is vital for visual processing and spatial awareness. Individuals may first appear with visual abnormalities and problems with spatial skills before experiencing broader cognitive deterioration.

Each variety of dementia involves specific obstacles for diagnosis, treatment, and caring. Advances in neuroimaging, biomarker studies, and understanding genetic variables contribute to continued efforts in detecting and managing these complicated disorders. Early identification and tailored care strategies are critical in increasing the quality of life and managing symptoms successfully for persons and their caregivers experiencing these varied kinds of dementia.

Causes and Risk Factors

Understanding the origins and risk factors of dementia is vital for creating prevention measures and therapies.

Causes of Dementia

Neurodegenerative Diseases: The most frequent cause of dementia is Alzheimer's disease, accounting for 60-80% of cases. Other neurodegenerative disorders include Parkinson's disease, Huntington's disease, and frontotemporal dementia. These disorders are distinguished by gradual brain cell destruction and loss.

Vascular Dementia: Strokes or other disorders that restrict or limit blood flow to the brain may cause vascular dementia. This kind of dementia originates from brain injury owing to cerebrovascular disorders, such as atherosclerosis or hemorrhages.

Mixed Dementia: In certain situations, people may display symptoms of more than one kind of dementia concurrently, such as Alzheimer's disease mixed with vascular dementia.

Other Medical illnesses: Certain illnesses may contribute to dementia-like symptoms, including infections (including HIV), persistent drinking, extended drug use, brain tumors, and vitamin deficiencies.

Risk Factors for Dementia

Age: The most significant major risk factor for dementia is age. The probability of having dementia grows considerably as individuals grow older, significantly beyond the age of 65.

Genetics: Family history and genetics have a role in dementia risk. Specific genes, such as the APOE ε4 allele, are connected with an increased risk of Alzheimer's disease.

Cardiovascular Health: Conditions that impact the heart and blood arteries, such as hypertension, high cholesterol, and diabetes, might raise the risk of dementia. Maintaining cardiovascular health is crucial to minimizing this risk.

Lifestyle Factors: Lifestyle decisions may strongly effect dementia risk. Smoking, heavy alcohol intake, physical inactivity, and poor nutrition are connected with more significant risks. Conversely, a healthy lifestyle, including regular exercise and a balanced diet, may help decrease these risks.

Mental and Social Engagement: Cognitive inactivity and social isolation might raise the risk of dementia. Protective factors include Engaging in intellectually engaging activities, maintaining social relationships, and lifelong learning.

Head traumas: A history of severe or recurrent head traumas might enhance the chance of acquiring dementia. This is especially pertinent for persons active in contact sports or those who have endured considerable trauma.

Depression and Psychological Health: Depression, mainly if it arises in mid-life or is recurring, has been related to an increased risk of dementia.

By knowing these causes and risk factors, people and healthcare professionals may better concentrate on preventive and early intervention measures to manage and lessen the burden of dementia.

Symptoms and Stages

Dementia symptoms vary but usually include memory loss, trouble finding words, and issues with problem-solving. Individuals may fail to execute familiar activities, display confusion about time or location, and suffer changes in mood or behavior. As dementia advances, these symptoms intensify, disrupting everyday living severely. For instance, someone with dementia could forget recent events or names of known individuals, have difficulties understanding discussions, or lose stuff often.

Stages of Dementia:

Dementia typically progresses through several stages:

Early Stage: Symptoms may be modest and easily disregarded in the early stages. Memory gaps could occur, such as forgetting previous conversations or occurrences, although persons can frequently still operate independently. They may tend to retreat from social or stressful circumstances to avoid shame.

Middle Stage: As dementia grows, symptoms become more visible and disruptive. Memory loss accelerates, making remembering personal history or identifying relatives and friends difficult. Communication issues worsen, with difficulty finding the correct words or following discussions. Individuals may require support with everyday duties like dressing or handling money. Behavioral changes, such as agitation or wandering, might also arise.

Late Stage: In the late stage of dementia, people need substantial care and assistance. Memory loss is significant; people may no longer recognize close family members or comprehend their surroundings. Communication is highly hindered frequently restricted to nonverbal displays. Physical capacities decrease, making movement and self-care difficult without support. Behavioral symptoms like hostility or agitation may increase, needing specialist treatment.

Throughout these phases, dementia affects each person individually, impacted by variables including underlying causes (such as Alzheimer's disease or vascular dementia) and specific health problems. Caregivers are critical in controlling symptoms, maintaining safety, and boosting the quality of life for persons with dementia.

Early identification by medical examination and monitoring of symptoms allows for prompt action and planning, including medication management, therapy, and support services. While dementia is degenerative and presently has no cure, recognizing its signs and phases helps families and caregivers offer appropriate care and support, providing dignity and comfort for persons afflicted by this complicated illness.

CHAPTER 2: DIAGNOSIS AND ASSESSMENT

Recognizing Early Signs

Recognizing early signs of dementia is critical for quick diagnosis and appropriate care of the illness. Dementia is a combination of symptoms affecting memory, reasoning, and social functions sufficiently enough to impair everyday life. Early identification allows for therapies that may decrease its course and enhance quality of life.

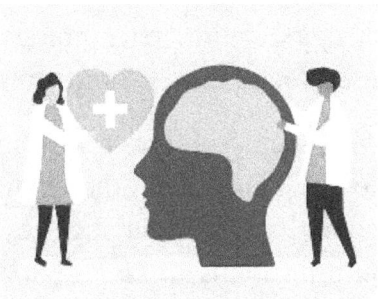

One of the early indicators of dementia is memory loss, which impairs everyday living. This goes beyond forgetting names or appointments infrequently; it entails losing freshly acquired knowledge, asking for the same information again, or depending on memory aides more regularly.

Another early symptom is difficulty in planning or addressing challenges. Individuals may struggle to follow a plan or work with numbers, such as managing funds or following a regular recipe. They may also face problems executing familiar chores at home, business, or leisure, leading to irritation or perplexity.

Changes in visual perception might also be informative. This could entail trouble calculating distances or identifying color contrasts, which might compromise driving skills or create issues with reading.

Additionally, persons with early dementia may find it challenging to follow or join a discussion. They could stop amid a sentence and not know how to continue or struggle with terminology, calling objects by the incorrect name or using ambiguous phrases.

Misplacing objects and being unable to retrace steps to locate them is another indicator. This is distinct from sometimes misplacing keys or spectacles; it entails putting items in strange locations and being unable to retrace steps to recover them.

Social disengagement and changes in mood or personality might potentially suggest early dementia. Individuals may become indifferent or disengaged from social events, professional initiatives, or hobbies they formerly liked. They may also experience mood swings or changes in personality, becoming confused, distrustful, scared, or nervous.

Recognizing these early indicators invites further investigation by a healthcare practitioner. Diagnosis typically entails a complete examination, including medical history, cognitive testing, physical exams, and occasionally brain imaging. Early diagnosis enables the adoption of methods to control symptoms, prepare for future care requirements, and access support resources. Family members and caregivers have a critical role in noticing and reporting these changes providing early intervention and support for those suffering from early stages of dementia.

Seeking Medical Help

Among the most essential steps in treating and understanding dementia is to seek medical attention. A collection of symptoms known as dementia impairs thinking, memory, and social skills to the point that they become disruptive to day-to-day functioning. Early identification and intervention are crucial for patients and their caregivers to have better quality of life and to better manage their symptoms.

First and first, it's critical to identify dementia symptoms. A few examples of these include memory loss that interferes with day-to-day functioning, difficulties organizing or solving problems, difficulty finishing familiar tasks, disorientation regarding time and location, difficulties comprehending visual images and spatial relationships, new challenges with words when speaking or writing, losing things and being unable to trace steps back, diminished or poor judgment, withdrawal from job or social activities, as well as changes in mood and conduct. As soon as these symptoms are seen, it is imperative to seek medical attention.

Getting medical assistance for dementia usually entails going to a specialist who can provide a comprehensive assessment, such as a neurologist or primary care physician. To rule out further potential reasons for cognitive decline, this assessment often consists of a review of medical history, mental tests, physical exams, and sometimes imaging tests like MRI or CT scans. The healthcare practitioner may also inquire about daily schedules, medication use, and any recent behavioral or cognitive changes.

After a diagnosis, medical professionals can advise on available treatments, including prescription drugs to control symptoms, counseling to improve communication skills through speech or cognitive behavioral therapy, or suggestions for lifestyle changes to improve general wellbeing. Early intervention not only aids in managing symptoms but also makes it feasible to put measures in place that will promote independence and everyday functioning for as long as possible.

In addition to medical care, dementia support programs may be beneficial. These services might include patient and caregiver support groups, educational courses on dementia and its treatment, and connections to neighborhood resources that help with everyday tasks or provide caregivers a break from caring for their loved ones.

Diagnostic Tests and Tools

Cognitive Assessments

Cognitive assessments for dementia are crucial instruments used by healthcare professionals to evaluate and diagnose cognitive deficits associated with different kinds of dementia, like Alzheimer's disease. These evaluations comprise a variety of tests meant to assess several areas of mental functioning, including memory, attention, linguistic ability, and problem-solving capabilities. These examinations aim to identify early indicators of dementia, monitor disease development, and aid in formulating suitable treatment plans and strategies.

One of the most regularly utilized cognitive testing methods is the Mini-Mental State Examination (MMSE). This short exam measures various cognitive areas via memory recall, orientation to time and location, and basic arithmetic computations. The scores obtained from the MMSE may reflect the level of cognitive impairment and assist in distinguishing between normal aging and dementia-related cognitive decline.

Another extensively employed examination is the Montreal Cognitive examination (MoCA), which thoroughly evaluates cognitive skills such as visuospatial ability, executive functions, and verbal fluency. The MoCA is especially sensitive to mild cognitive impairment (MCI), a condition that commonly precedes dementia and needs regular monitoring.

In addition to these standardized exams, healthcare practitioners may perform additional customized evaluations based on the patient's symptoms and medical history. For instance, examinations of language skills, such as the Boston Naming Test or the Controlled Oral Word Association Test (COWAT), may be used to examine language deficits often linked with particular kinds of dementia, such as frontotemporal dementia.

The process of performing cognitive evaluations for dementia entails providing tests and evaluating findings within the context of the patient's general health and medical history. Factors such as education level, cultural background, and comorbidities might impact test performance and must be addressed for appropriate diagnosis and treatment planning.

Cognitive evaluations are diagnostic tools that serve as baseline measurements for monitoring illness development and assessing the efficiency of therapies, such as medication and mental rehabilitation programs. Regular evaluation helps healthcare practitioners change treatment strategies properly and give vital support to patients and their families throughout the illness.

Imaging Tests

Imaging tests serve a significant role in the diagnosis and treatment of dementia, a degenerative neurological disorder marked by cognitive loss. These tests employ modern medical imaging technology to see the brain's structure, function, and blood flow, supporting physicians in identifying the underlying causes of dementia and guiding treatment options.

One of the most regularly utilized imaging methods is magnetic resonance imaging (MRI). MRI gives comprehensive pictures of the brain's structure, enabling clinicians to spot alterations such as shrinkage in particular areas linked with distinct forms of dementia. For instance, Alzheimer's disease, the most prevalent type of dementia, generally reveals recognizable patterns of brain shrinkage evident on MRI scans. These photos let medics discriminate between distinct kinds of dementia and follow disease development over time.

Another excellent imaging technology is positron emission tomography (PET). PET scans give functional information about brain activity and metabolism using radioactive tracers highlighting brain regions impacted by dementia-related alterations. In Alzheimer's disease, PET scans may indicate the deposition of beta-amyloid plaques, a characteristic of the disorder. Additionally, PET scans may examine glucose metabolism, which is typically changed in patients with dementia, allowing them to discriminate between various kinds of dementia and track therapy responses.

Single-photon emission computed tomography (SPECT) is another imaging technique for dementia diagnosis. Like PET, SPECT scans give information on cerebral blood flow and brain activity patterns. SPECT imaging is especially effective in detecting regions of diminished blood flow, which might suggest areas of neuronal injury or dysfunction associated with dementia. This approach assists in early diagnosis and may help predict individuals' cognitive impairment trajectory.

Advanced imaging methods, such as functional MRI (fMRI) and diffusion tensor imaging (DTI), give further insights into brain activity and connectivity in persons with dementia. fMRI monitors blood flow variations associated with brain activity, helping map cognitive skills like memory and language. DTI, on the other hand, evaluates the brain's white matter pathways, finding anomalies in connection that may lead to cognitive impairment

Laboratory Tests

Laboratory testing is significant in diagnosing dementia, supporting doctors in verifying concerns prompted by clinical assessments and symptoms. While dementia itself cannot be reliably diagnosed by lab testing alone, these studies are crucial in ruling out other illnesses that may resemble dementia symptoms and in identifying probable underlying causes. Here are major laboratory tests typically utilized in the diagnosis process:

Blood Tests are critical for monitoring general health and ruling out disorders that might influence cognitive function. Tests often include a complete blood count (CBC) to screen for infections or anemia, thyroid function tests to identify thyroid abnormalities, and vitamin B12 levels since deficits may lead to cognitive impairment.

Metabolic Panels: Comprehensive metabolic panels (CMP) and basic metabolic panels (BMP) assist in testing kidney and liver function, electrolyte levels, and glucose levels. Abnormalities in these regions may disrupt brain function and lead to cognitive impairment.

Lipid Profile: High cholesterol levels may raise the risk of vascular dementia; lipid profiles are commonly used to examine cardiovascular health and possible risk factors.

Genetic Testing: While not a typical aspect of diagnosis, genetic testing may detect genes related to early-onset familial types of dementia, like Alzheimer's disease. This information may inform prognosis and influence family planning choices.

Cerebrospinal Fluid (CSF) Analysis: In select circumstances, a lumbar puncture may be conducted to examine CSF for biomarkers linked with certain kinds of dementia, like Alzheimer's. Elevated tau protein and lower amyloid-beta levels in CSF may support a diagnosis of Alzheimer's.

Neuroimaging: Though not a laboratory test per se, neuroimaging methods like MRI or CT scans are vital for identifying structural brain abnormalities, such as tumors, strokes, or brain atrophy, which may contribute to dementia symptoms.

Neuropsychological Testing: While primarily a clinical examination, neuropsychological tests assist in examining cognitive processes, including memory, attention, and language abilities. Results may complement lab results and assist in detecting particular kinds of dementia.

Laboratory testing in dementia diagnosis is crucial in eliminating reversible causes of cognitive loss and giving supporting evidence for certain kinds of dementia. They contribute to a complete diagnostic strategy incorporating clinical history, physical examination, and imaging investigations to establish an accurate diagnosis. Effective treatment and management methods focus on understanding the underlying reasons and adapting care appropriately, making these tests crucial in diagnosing dementia.

Understanding the Diagnosis

Understanding the diagnosis of dementia includes traversing a complicated environment of symptoms, evaluations, and medical procedures. Dementia is a collection of cognitive illnesses defined by a deterioration in memory, thinking, and other mental processes that interfere with everyday living. It's vital to clarify how healthcare professionals diagnose dementia to provide prompt intervention and support for patients and their families.

Diagnosing dementia typically starts with a complete medical history review and a full physical and neurological examination. Healthcare practitioners depend on these early measures to discover any underlying disorders or drugs that might contribute to cognitive impairment. Next, they typically do cognitive exams and screenings to check memory, linguistic ability, problem-solving capabilities, and attention span. These tests help create a baseline for mental performance and identify any impairments that may suggest dementia.

Imaging studies, such as CT scans or MRI scans, are routinely performed to rule out other possible reasons for cognitive loss, such as brain tumors, strokes, or fluid accumulation. These scans give precise pictures of the brain's structure, assisting in diagnosing anomalies or changes linked with dementia.

In addition to clinical examinations, laboratory testing may be undertaken to check thyroid function, vitamin B12 levels, and other metabolic parameters potentially impacting brain health. These tests aid in eliminating reversible sources of cognitive impairment, ensuring that the diagnosis of dementia is accurate and complete.

A significant element of dementia diagnosis requires evaluating the patient's history and tracking their symptoms over time. Healthcare practitioners commonly involve family members or caregivers in this approach to get insight into the development and course of cognitive loss. Family members' viewpoints might give valuable information regarding changes in behavior, memory lapses, or difficulty with everyday tasks that may not be readily evident during professional exams.

Communicating the Diagnosis to the Family

Communicating a dementia diagnosis to family members is a sensitive and emotionally charged undertaking that demands compassion, clarity, and empathy. Dementia, a degenerative disorder impairing cognitive ability, may have tremendous consequences on both the afflicted people and their loved ones. Effectively communicating this diagnosis entails many critical aspects to guarantee understanding and support within the family.

Firstly, time plays a critical role in conveying such news. It is ideal to arrange a time when all relevant family members may be present and in a comfortable location conducive to open conversation. This helps establish an environment where emotions may be shared, and questions can be answered without excessive pressure or distraction.

Clarity in communication is vital. Using primary language everyone can comprehend helps demystify the disease and its effects. It's crucial to convey accurate information regarding dementia, including its symptoms, development, and possible therapies or management options. This empowers family members with information, eliminating uncertainty and anxiety.

Empathy and emotional support are equally vital throughout this discourse. Recognizing and accepting the emotional effect of the diagnosis on family members develops a feeling of connection and solidarity. They encouraged free expression of emotions, whether grief, worry, or perplexity, acknowledging their experiences and improving family relationships.

Furthermore, integrating family members in decision-making processes may help lessen emotions of powerlessness or isolation. Discussing future care planning and practical issues together allows for collective participation and ensures everyone feels included and valued in assisting their loved one with dementia.

Educating family members on how they may give physical aid and emotional support can also be valuable. This may involve learning about caring practices, services accessible in the community, and how to communicate effectively with someone facing dementia-related issues.

Lastly, continual communication is crucial. Dementia is a degenerative disorder, and its influence may develop over time. Regular updates and conversations about changes in the loved one's health, treatment choices, and family duties ensure that everyone stays aware and active in giving the best possible care and support.

CHAPTER 3: TREATMENT AND MANAGEMENT

Medical Treatments
Medications

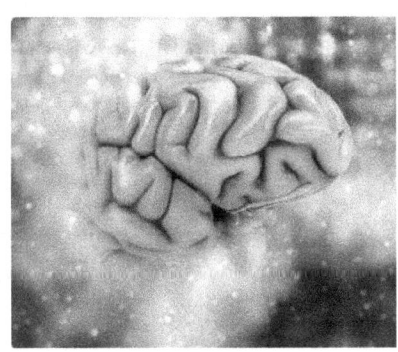

Dementia has no cure, but drugs may help control symptoms. These drugs fall into two primary categories: cholinesterase inhibitors and memantine.

Cholinesterase inhibitors are a significant therapy for Alzheimer's disease and several other dementias. These medications act by boosting the levels of acetylcholine, a neurotransmitter important in memory and judgment. The most often prescribed cholinesterase inhibitors include:

Donepezil (Aricept): Approved for all stages of Alzheimer's disease, donepezil is given once daily. It may enhance cognition and behavior by improving communication between nerve cells.

Rivastigmine (Exelon): Available as a tablet, liquid, or patch, rivastigmine is authorized for mild to moderate Alzheimer's and Parkinson's disease dementia. It acts similarly to donepezil but must be taken twice daily or administered as a patch once daily.

Galantamine (Razadyne): Used for mild to severe Alzheimer's, galantamine is administered twice daily. It enhances acetylcholine levels and activates nicotinic receptors, boosting cognitive function.

These medications may assist with symptoms like memory loss, confusion, and difficulty with thinking and reasoning, but they do not halt the course of the illness. Side effects may include nausea, vomiting, lack of appetite, and increased frequency of bowel motions.

Memantine (Namenda) is another medicine authorized for moderate to severe Alzheimer's disease. Unlike cholinesterase inhibitors, memantine modulates the function of glutamate, another neurotransmitter important in learning and memory. It is commonly used in tandem with a cholinesterase inhibitor. Memantine may aid in increasing memory, attention, reason, language, and the capacity to do basic activities. Side effects may include dizziness, headache, disorientation, and constipation.

Additionally, combination medications like Namzaric, which contains donepezil and memantine, are available. This combination may help control symptoms in people with moderate to severe Alzheimer's disease more successfully than either medicine alone.

While these medications help relieve specific symptoms and enhance quality of life, they do not change the disease's underlying pathophysiology. Ongoing research is focused on developing more effective medicines that can reduce or halt the course of dementia. In the meantime, drugs, together with supportive therapy and lifestyle adjustments, remain the cornerstone of dementia care.

Non-pharmacological Treatments

Non-pharmacological treatments for dementia cover several techniques that concentrate on enhancing the quality of life for patients without the use of drugs. These treatments are beneficial since they often come with fewer side effects and may be tailored to match the unique demands of each individual. Let's dig into these therapies in further detail:

Cognitive Stimulation Therapy (CST)

Cognitive Stimulation Therapy (CST) is a non-pharmacological intervention meant to enhance mental function and quality of life for those living with dementia. It incorporates organized sessions of themed activities and conversations performed in small groups, often guided by a certified facilitator. CST seeks to excite and engage multiple cognitive processes such as memory, attention, language, and problem-solving abilities, which may diminish with dementia development.

The treatment is founded on the principles of neuroplasticity, which imply that the brain can rearrange and generate new neural connections in response to learning and experience, even amid neurodegenerative disorders like dementia. By offering controlled and purposeful activities, CST strives to build cognitive reserve, possibly slowing mental decline and boosting general well-being.

Sessions frequently involve a range of activities such as word games, recollection exercises, puzzles, and creative assignments, all adapted to the skills and interests of the participants. The group structure offers cognitive stimulation and stimulates social contact and emotional support, which are vital for preserving a sense of connection and minimizing feelings of isolation typically experienced by those with dementia.

Research on CST has shown encouraging results, including increased cognitive function, mood, and communication skills among participants. It is considered a person-centered approach, concentrating on the individual's strengths and preferences rather than weaknesses. CST is often provided over many weeks or months, with sessions done frequently to optimize its advantages.

Reminiscence Therapy

Reminiscence therapy is a therapeutic strategy commonly utilized in the treatment of dementia, seeking to increase the quality of life for persons living with cognitive disorders. It includes the discussion of prior experiences, events, and personal recollections, typically encouraged by discussions, images, music, or familiar items from the person's past. The treatment harnesses the intact long-term memory of dementia patients, providing comfort, validation, and emotional connection.

Central to recollection therapy is its potential to create happy feelings and boost mood by tapping into remembering meaningful life experiences. Studies show that participating in reminiscing helps lessen agitation, anxiety, and depressed symptoms typically linked with dementia. Creating a feeling of continuity and identity helps people keep a link to their personal history and identity despite cognitive deterioration.

Moreover, remembrance therapy may function as a social activity, increasing connection and communication between dementia patients, caregivers, and family members. This social involvement is vital in fighting emotions of isolation and loneliness that typically accompany dementia. Through shared reminiscence, it generates opportunities for meaningful connections and develops relationships.

From a neurological standpoint, recollection therapy activates several brain areas related to memory recall and emotional processing. It might slow down cognitive decline by strengthening neuronal circuits involved in memory retrieval. This mental stimulation is good not just for memory retention but also for general cognitive performance.

In practice, reminiscence therapy sessions are adjusted to individual preferences and capabilities, guaranteeing a personalized and happy experience. Caregivers and healthcare professionals are critical in organizing these sessions, offering a supportive setting that facilitates remembering and emotional expression.

Validation Therapy

Validation Therapy is a caring approach to dementia care that focuses on sympathetic communication and emotional validation rather than factual correction. Developed by Naomi Feil in the 1960s, this treatment tries to connect with patients with dementia emotionally, accepting and supporting their emotions, memories, and experiences, even if they do not fit with reality.

Central to Validation Therapy is the concept that persons with dementia typically suffer confusion and discomfort owing to their deteriorating cognitive ability. Instead of questioning their views or seeking to bring them back to reality, Validation Therapy urges caregivers to join their world, validate their feelings, and provide comfort and reassurance. This technique helps minimize emotions of anxiety, irritation, and agitation in dementia patients by promoting a sense of understanding and acceptance.

Validation Therapy approaches include active listening, mirroring feelings, utilizing soothing gestures, and reminiscing about prior events to create a supportive atmosphere. Caregivers are educated to affirm the person's emotions and recollections, regardless of their correctness, which may enhance the patient's general well-being and quality of life.

Research on Validation Therapy reveals that it helps strengthen communication between caregivers and dementia patients, resulting in fewer behavioral symptoms and greater emotional connection. By emphasizing emotional affirmation rather than cognitive correction, this method respects the individual's dignity and agency while establishing a more positive caring relationship.

Music Therapy

Music therapy is an increasingly popular treatment for patients with dementia, delivering considerable emotional, cognitive, and social advantages. This therapeutic technique uses the power of music to engage and excite the brain, giving a non-pharmacological alternative to promote quality of life.

Research suggests that music therapy helps improve several symptoms of dementia, such as agitation, melancholy, and anxiety. Music's rhythm and melody may stimulate memories and emotions, enabling people to reconnect with their past and express themselves. Familiar songs may evoke autobiographical memories, producing a feeling of continuity and identity.

Cognitive gains are also noticeable, with music therapy improving language skills, concentration, and executive function. The organized form of music, notably its repeating rhythms, may aid in increasing attention and cognitive processing. Furthermore, group music therapy sessions enhance social contact, lowering feelings of isolation and loneliness that are typical in dementia patients.

The physical effects of music therapy should not be disregarded. Engaging in hobbies like singing or playing instruments helps boost motor skills and coordination. For certain patients, these activities might help improve calm and lessen agitation.

Implementing music therapy entails specific treatments according to the individual's tastes and background. Certified music therapists examine the patient's requirements and arrange sessions involving listening to music, singing, playing instruments, or even writing music. This individualized approach guarantees that the treatment connects strongly with the individual, boosting its therapeutic potential.

Physical Exercise

Physical exercise has emerged as a viable non-pharmacological method for controlling dementia. Dementia, an illness marked by a deterioration in memory, reasoning, behavior, and the capacity to conduct daily tasks, affects millions worldwide. Research increasingly shows that regular physical exercise might enhance cognitive function and overall quality of life for persons with dementia.

One of the primary advantages of physical exercise in dementia therapy is its potential to enhance brain health. Exercise increases the production of chemicals that encourage the development of brain cells and new connections between cells, a process known as neuroplasticity. This may help alleviate some of the cognitive deterioration associated with dementia by perhaps slowing down the course of the condition.

Moreover, physical exercise has been demonstrated to improve cardiovascular health, increase mood, and lower stress and anxiety levels, all of which are good for persons with dementia and their caregivers. Regular exercise routines, such as walking, swimming, or even basic stretching exercises, may help boost physical strength and balance, minimizing the chance of falls and accompanying injuries, which are significant concerns among dementia patients.

Physical exercise is a diverse intervention that can be customized to individual requirements and skills. It may be customized to different stages of dementia, from early to advanced, and can be conducted in various settings, including at home or in specialist care facilities. Even brief periods of exercise many times a week have been demonstrated to impact cognitive performance and general well-being positively.

Art Therapy

Art therapy has emerged as a viable treatment for those suffering from dementia, giving a creative and expressive outlet that may considerably boost their quality of life. Dementia, a progressive neurological condition, generally leads to cognitive decline, memory loss, and behavioral abnormalities, harming both patients and their caretakers. Art therapy involves many types of creative expression, such as painting, sketching, sculpture, and collage-making, to engage dementia patients in meaningful activities that boost cognitive processes and emotional well-being.

One of the primary advantages of art therapy is its ability to transcend verbal communication hurdles typically faced by people living with dementia. Artistic interests assist individuals to express themselves non-verbally, tapping into memories, emotions, and sensory experiences that may otherwise be difficult to explain. This treatment may relieve tension, anxiety, and sadness while fostering relaxation and achievement.

Moreover, participating in creative undertakings might increase cognitive capabilities by activating diverse parts of the brain. Studies have shown that art therapy may improve memory recall, problem-solving ability, and general mental flexibility in dementia patients. It offers a controlled and secure setting where people may explore their creativity without fear of criticism, boosting self-esteem and confidence.

Art therapy enhances social relationships and communication skills, fostering interaction between patients, caregivers, and therapists. Group sessions may establish a supportive community where people share experiences, memories, and emotions via art, increasing a sense of belonging and minimizing feelings of loneliness.

Environmental Modifications

Environmental modifications for dementia therapies entail altering physical environments to increase the well-being and quality of life for persons with dementia. These improvements attempt to provide a supportive atmosphere that reduces confusion, agitation, and stress while fostering independence and safety.

One essential part is ensuring the environment is secure and readily navigated. This involves eliminating dangers such as loose carpets, debris, or furniture restricting routes. Clear routes with excellent lighting and color contrast may help folks recognize various regions and travel more comfortably. Installing grab bars and handrails in essential areas like toilets and corridors helps minimize the danger of falls.

Creating a peaceful and pleasant environment is vital. This may be done by limiting noise levels, utilizing relaxing hues like light blues or greens, and eliminating patterns that may induce confusion. Natural light and access to outdoor places may also have therapeutic effects, providing a connection to nature that can decrease agitation and enhance mood.

Adapting furniture and fittings for comfort and ease of use is vital. Choosing comfortable and supportive seats helps folks stay comfortable for longer durations. Labeling drawers, cabinets, and rooms with clear signs or images may assist with orienting and memory recall. Additionally, utilizing familiar and vital things may recall happy memories and bring comfort.

Technology may play a crucial influence in environmental alterations. Smart home devices may automate functions like changing lights or monitoring temperatures, boosting convenience and safety. GPS monitoring systems may assist in preventing wandering, a significant issue for those with dementia, offering peace of mind to caretakers.

Sensory Stimulation

Sensory stimulation is an emerging strategy in dementia therapy, aiming to increase the quality of life for patients with cognitive impairments. This treatment method includes engaging the senses—sight, hearing, touch, taste, and smell—to create good emotional reactions and promote mental functioning.

Visual stimulation includes activities such as viewing colorful films, gazing at family pictures, or enjoying beautiful vistas, which may aid in evoking memories and delivering a relaxing impact. Auditory stimulation, such as listening to music, natural sounds, or familiar voices, may generate feelings and sometimes even induce verbal communication in non-verbal patients.

Tactile stimulation involves handling textured materials, gardening, or participating in basic crafts. These exercises may assist in developing motor abilities and bring comfort via familiar physical feelings. Taste and smell stimulation may be performed by culinary activities, eating favorite meals, or using aromatherapy. Familiar tastes and fragrances may trigger memories and emotions, offering comfort and familiarity.

One notable advantage of sensory stimulation is its capacity to alleviate agitation and anxiety, especially in dementia patients. By engaging the senses, these activities may create a more soothing atmosphere, lowering behavioral concerns and boosting overall mood. Additionally, sensory stimulation may increase social connection since many activities can be done in group settings, establishing a sense of community and minimizing feelings of loneliness.

Implementing sensory stimulation in dementia care involves an individualized approach, considering the individual's preferences and background to ensure the activities are relevant and pleasurable. Caregivers and healthcare personnel play a significant role in arranging these activities and evaluating the patient's reactions to adapt the treatment appropriately.

Social Engagement

Social engagement is widely acknowledged as essential in treating and managing dementia. Interaction with others may significantly boost the quality of life for persons with dementia, giving emotional support, cerebral stimulation, and chances for physical exercise. Engaging socially can lessen feelings of loneliness and sadness, which are frequent among persons with dementia, therefore increasing general well-being.

One significant advantage of social involvement is its stimulation of the brain. Group discussions, games, and even simple talks may assist in sustaining cognitive function. These interactions stimulate patients to exercise their memory and problem-solving abilities, which may halt cognitive loss. Additionally, social activities generally entail physical mobility, whether dancing, strolling, or engaging in group exercises, vital for sustaining physical health.

Programs meant to enhance social interaction may be adapted to meet the interests and skills of persons with dementia. For example, music therapy groups, painting courses, and gardening clubs allow patients to interact with others while participating in meaningful activities. These programs promote social connection and provide a feeling of purpose and success.

Family participation is also vital to social engagement for people with dementia. Encouraging family members to engage in events and keep frequent contact may help establish emotional attachments and offer a support network for the patient and caretakers. This engagement helps keep patients linked to their loved ones, promoting a feeling of belonging and continuity.

Aromatherapy

Aromatherapy, an alternative treatment involving essential oils produced from plants, provides several advantages for patients with dementia. These essential oils are usually supplied by inhalation, massage, or baths and are thought to improve mood, cognitive performance, and physical well-being.

How Aromatherapy Works

It is believed that essential oils may change the brain's limbic system, which controls emotions, behavior, and long-term memory. When breathed, the smell molecules from the essential oils go down the nasal passages and into the brain, where they may have a relaxing or energizing impact. Varied oils are connected with varied therapeutic benefits, making aromatherapy a diverse treatment approach.

Common Essential Oils Used in Dementia Care

Lavender: Known for its relaxing effects, lavender oil is widely used to decrease anxiety agitation and induce sleep. Its pleasant aroma may help consumers feel more relaxed and less anxious.

Rosemary: This oil is typically used to increase memory and attention. It provides a stimulating impact that may aid in boosting cognitive function and attentiveness.

Peppermint: Peppermint oil is stimulating and may help relieve symptoms of weariness and despair. It is also recognized for its ability to promote attention and mental clarity.

Bergamot: With its uplifting and invigorating aroma, bergamot oil may help enhance mood and ease symptoms of anxiety and despair. It is especially effective in establishing a more happy emotional state.

Lemon Balm (Melissa): Known for its relaxing and anti-anxiety effects, lemon balm oil may help decrease agitation and produce a feeling of relaxation and well-being.

Ylang-Ylang: This oil is recognized for its soothing and sedative characteristics, effectively lowering stress and facilitating better sleep.

Methods of Application

Inhalation: Essential oils may be dispersed into the air using an essential oil diffuser. This approach enables the smell molecules to be breathed, giving a rapid and efficient way to enjoy the advantages of aromatherapy. Personal inhalers or just pouring a few drops of oil on a handkerchief may also be utilized for direct inhalation.

Topical Application: Essential oils may be diluted with a carrier oil (such as coconut or jojoba oil) and administered to the skin via massage. This approach combines the therapeutic effects of both touch and fragrance, promoting relaxation and lowering physical stress.

Baths: Adding a few drops of essential oil to a warm bath may produce a peaceful and therapeutic experience. The mix of warm water and fragrant oils helps to relax the muscles, quiet the mind, and boost overall mood.

Benefits of Aromatherapy for Dementia

Reduction of Anxiety and Agitation: Aromatherapy may help decrease anxiety and agitation, frequent symptoms in patients with dementia. The relaxing properties of particular essential oils may generate a more serene and relaxed mood, making it more straightforward for people to deal with their surroundings.

Improvement in Sleep: Sleep difficulties are typical in people with dementia. Essential oils such as lavender and ylang-ylang help improve sleep by encouraging calm and minimizing nightly awakenings.

Enhanced Mood and Emotional Well-being: Essential oils like bergamot and lemon balm help boost mood and lessen symptoms of despair. Aromatherapy is a non-invasive technique to increase mental well-being and create a more cheerful environment.

Cognitive Benefits: Oils such as rosemary and peppermint may stimulate the mind, enhancing memory, attention, and mental performance. These advantages may help folks stay more attentive and engaged.

Reduction in Physical Symptoms: Aromatherapy may also help reduce physical symptoms such as headaches, muscular pain, and digestive difficulties. The comprehensive aspect of this therapy targets both mental and physical well-being.

Precautions and Considerations

While aromatherapy has numerous advantages, utilizing essential oils safely and correctly is crucial. Essential oils should always be diluted before topical use to prevent skin irritation. It is also essential to consider any allergies or sensitivities the person may have to various smells. Consulting with a healthcare expert or a qualified aromatherapist helps guarantee that aromatherapy is utilized safely and efficiently.

Managing Co-existing Conditions

Managing dementia in individuals with co-existing diseases demands a thorough and individualized approach to caring and treatment. Dementia, a degenerative neurological ailment, typically coexists with numerous other health concerns, such as cardiovascular disease, diabetes, and depression, complicating both diagnosis and care. The key to successful care is treating each ailment holistically while considering their interaction and influence on the individual's general health and cognitive function.

Firstly, a comprehensive examination by healthcare specialists is needed to identify all current illnesses and their unique consequences for dementia treatment. This involves examining cognitive performance, physical health, drug regimens, and psychological well-being. A tailored care plan may then be devised, incorporating therapies for each illness to enhance results while limiting possible interactions or side effects from many drugs.

Medication management is especially crucial since patients with dementia and co-existing diseases sometimes need many medicines. Careful monitoring and occasional assessments by healthcare practitioners ensure that drugs are appropriate, effective, and safe. Non-pharmacological therapies also play a crucial role, such as lifestyle alterations, dietary adjustments, and physical exercise targeted to both dementia and co-existing illnesses.

Support from caregivers and family members is crucial in treating dementia and its co-existing diseases. Education regarding the illnesses, their development, and caring practices may allow caregivers to offer more excellent assistance while preserving their well-being. Regular contact with healthcare experts enables revisions to the treatment plan as required, particularly since symptoms may develop over time.

Lastly, providing a supportive atmosphere that increases quality of life is vital. This involves establishing a secure and familiar living place, fostering social connections, and giving chances for meaningful activities. Managing dementia with co-existing diseases requires a coordinated effort involving healthcare providers, caregivers, and persons seeking to maintain cognitive function, control symptoms, and maximize overall health and well-being.

CHAPTER 4: DAILY LIVING AND CAREGIVING

Creating a Safe and Comfortable Environment

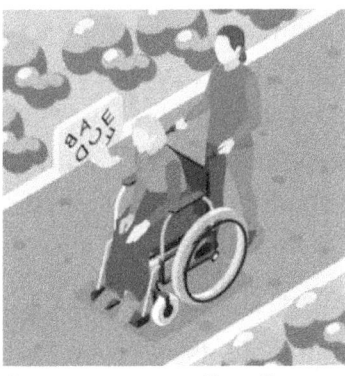

Creating a safe and pleasant environment for dementia patients entails many critical aspects to guarantee their well-being and quality of life. Central to this endeavor is changing the physical environment to decrease confusion, encourage independence, and increase overall safety.

Firstly, it's vital to simplify the environment by minimizing clutter and unneeded goods that might be confusing or overpowering. Clear routes and well-defined zones may help avoid accidents and reduce anxiety. Labeling drawers, cabinets, and rooms with clear signs or images assists with orienting and fosters independence.

Secondly, maintaining appropriate illumination throughout the room is vital. Dim illumination may induce confusion and increase the risk of falls. Installing bright, non-glare lighting fixtures may increase vision and assist in preserving the patient's circadian cycles, enabling improved sleep habits.

Moreover, safety changes such as putting handrails in corridors and restrooms, using non-slip mats, and fastening carpets help avoid falls and injuries. Furniture should be designed to assist simple navigation and offer pleasant sitting spaces that encourage relaxation and social interaction.

Additionally, keeping a peaceful and soothing ambiance by using familiar and comfortable things, such as photographs, beloved books, or music, may stimulate happy memories and minimize tension. A regular schedule with planned activities may also create a feeling of security and purpose.

Lastly, constant appraisal of the environment and its adjustments is crucial since the patient's demands and abilities may vary. Consulting with healthcare experts, caregivers, and occupational therapists may offer significant insights and ideas for further strengthening the environment's appropriateness.

By stressing safety, simplicity, comfort, and familiarity in the surroundings, caregivers and loved ones may dramatically enhance the quality of life for dementia patients, creating a feeling of security and well-being among the obstacles given by the disease.

Daily Care Routines

Caring for a dementia patient involves a planned approach to daily routines involving personal cleanliness, clothing and grooming, nutrition, and meals. Each of these qualities is vital for sustaining physical health and developing a feeling of dignity and well-being in the person.

Personal Hygiene

Personal hygiene is essential in dementia care, preserving the patient's comfort and health. Daily routines should involve aiding the person with chores such as bathing, dental care, and toileting. It's crucial to handle these activities with compassion and respect since dementia may lead the individual to feel confused or irritated.

When assisting with bathing, it's beneficial to establish a warm, peaceful atmosphere to alleviate anxiety. Using soft, non-slip mats and proper bathing aids may increase safety. Communicating correctly and offering step-by-step assistance might make the patient feel more safe. Incorporating relaxing music or familiar fragrances might provide a more enjoyable experience for folks who may avoid showering.

Oral care should be conducted routinely to avoid dental disorders and preserve general health. Gentle reminders and showing suitable brushing methods might promote participation. Similarly, aiding with toileting requires patience and understanding, ensuring the person's dignity and privacy are maintained throughout.

Dressing and Grooming

Dressing and grooming routines should be reduced to meet the cognitive problems of dementia. Choosing comfortable, easy-to-manage outfits may foster independence while lowering frustration. Opting for clothing with fewer buttons or zippers and employing elastic waistbands may simplify dressing.

Providing precise alternatives rather than open-ended questions might make the patient feel more controlled. For example, placing up two wardrobe alternatives helps children to participate in decision-making without feeling overwhelmed. Offering help as required, such as moving arms through sleeves or fastening fasteners, enhances their independence while ensuring they are correctly clothed for comfort and weather circumstances.

Grooming procedures like hair care and shaving should be handled calmly and gently. Using gentle motions and verbal prompts may aid the patient in doing these activities independently or with little assistance. Maintaining a routine and utilizing familiar grooming products may also help alleviate anxiety and uncertainty.

Nutrition and Mealtime

Proper nutrition is crucial for general health and well-being. Planning healthy meals and snacks that are pleasant and simple to consume promotes the patient's physical and cognitive wellness. Establishing regular meal times and maintaining a peaceful, distraction-free atmosphere may help decrease confusion and create a happy dining experience.

When cooking meals, consider the individual's food preferences and any unique nutritional requirements—offering familiar and delightful meals increases eating. Finger foods or utensils modified for better grasp might promote independence during meals. Monitoring the patient's eating habits and maintaining appropriate water throughout the day is crucial.

During mealtime, offering clear, basic directions and allowing sufficient time for eating helps prevent frustration. Engaging in casual conversation or playing soothing music may create a comfortable ambiance and help the patient eat quickly. Help cutting food or offering vocal reminders may enhance independence while maintaining safety.

Daily Routine Caregiving Approach

In everyday caring practices for dementia patients, consistency and compassion are crucial. Establishing a consistent routine helps minimize anxiety and uncertainty, offering a feeling of stability for the person. Communicating gently and utilizing non-verbal signals such as soft touches or visual hints may increase comprehension and cooperation.

Adapting routines to meet the person's evolving skills and preferences is vital. Flexibility enables caregivers to react to the individual's requirements while encouraging freedom and dignity. Regularly analyzing and altering caregiving tactics depending on the patient's reactions and behaviors ensures that their daily routines continue to fulfill their growing requirements.

By focusing on personal cleanliness, clothing and grooming, and nutrition and meals within a planned daily routine, caregivers may increase the quality of life for dementia patients. Each care component should be addressed with empathy, respect, and understanding of the person's strengths and problems. Through careful and regular caring techniques, caregivers may assist the individual's well-being and protect their dignity throughout the advancement of dementia.

Communication Strategies

Effective communication is crucial while caring for dementia patients, eliminating confusion and promoting their quality of life. Caregivers should use primary, plain language, speak gently, and keep eye contact to show comfort and comprehension. Non-verbal clues, such as gentle touch or facial expressions, may complement verbal communication, assisting in emotional connection and understanding. Patience is vital, leaving appropriate time for replies and avoiding hurrying talks. Repetition of information helps strengthen knowledge, while visual aids, such as images or written notes, assist with memory recall and everyday routines. Consistency in communication patterns and procedures promotes stability, fostering security and minimizing patient anxiety.

Activities and Engagement

Engaging People with dementia in meaningful activities is crucial for cognitive stimulation and emotional well-being. Activities should be adapted to the patient's interests and skills, guaranteeing fun and involvement. Hobbies such as listening to music, reminiscing about familiar things, or indulging in mild activities boost mental alertness and physical well-being. Structured activities, such as puzzles or crafts with simplified directions, foster a feeling of success and independence. Outdoor activities like brief walks or gardening, customized to the patient's mobility, give sensory stimulation and connection with nature. Regularly evaluating the patient's reaction to activities lets caregivers change and optimize engagement techniques. By concentrating on tailored activities that promote mental, physical, and emotional health, caregivers may enrich the everyday lives of dementia patients, establishing a supportive atmosphere that supports their well-being.

Managing Challenging Behaviors
Aggression and Agitation

Managing aggressiveness and agitation in dementia patients involves a holistic strategy focused on identifying and resolving the underlying reasons for these behaviors. Aggression typically develops from frustration, uncertainty, or an inability to communicate demands verbally. Caregivers should keep a relaxed attitude and avoid conflicts, instead choosing gentle redirection and reassurance. Establishing a consistent schedule and generating a relaxing atmosphere might assist in preventing escalation. Non-verbal communication, such as keeping eye contact and utilizing calming gestures, may also assist in de-escalating uncomfortable circumstances. Caregivers must focus on empathy and patience, obtaining help from healthcare experts when required to build specific tactics that provide a serene atmosphere.

Wandering

Wandering is a prevalent activity among dementia patients that presents substantial safety hazards, including becoming lost or hurt. Caregivers may apply numerous techniques to control wandering behaviors efficiently. Installing door alarms or employing GPS tracking devices may assist in monitoring movements and prevent straying outside the house. Creating a safe environment with closed doors or gates that need a code might help dissuade roaming. Engaging the patient in supervised activities that give excitement and purpose helps minimize restlessness and the drive to roam. Ensuring the surroundings are familiar and pleasant may also lessen the incidence of wandering episodes. Caregivers should engage with healthcare experts to uncover underlying reasons and design individualized therapies that promote safety and support.

Sleep Issues

Sleep difficulties, such as insomnia or frequent awakening throughout the night, are significant issues for dementia patients and their caregivers. Establishing a soothing nighttime ritual may encourage relaxation and increase sleep quality. Activities such as mild stretching or listening to peaceful music before bed might help notify the body that it's time to sleep. A sleep-conducive atmosphere with comfortable bedding, little noise, and limited light exposure may further boost sleep hygiene. Limiting caffeine consumption and maintaining regular physical exercise throughout the day may also help to healthier sleep patterns. Caregivers should speak with healthcare providers to rule out underlying medical issues or pharmaceutical side effects that may contribute to sleep difficulties. Exploring suitable sleep aids or supplements under medical advice may assist in managing sleep disorders while balancing possible advantages and hazards for the patient's general well-being.

CHAPTER 5: LEGAL AND FINANCIAL PLANNING

Understanding Legal Documents

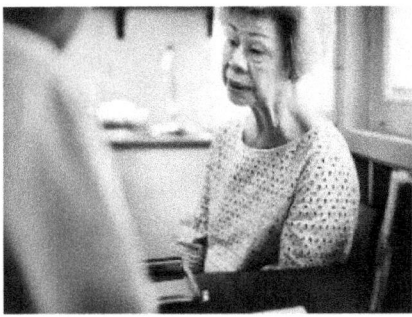

Legal papers play a crucial role in defending the rights and obligations of dementia caregivers. These papers, including Power of Attorney, Living Will, and Guardianship, are critical instruments that guarantee caretakers can adequately manage the affairs and well-being of those with dementia.

Power of Attorney

A Power of Attorney (POA) is a legal instrument that allows a chosen caregiver or agent to make financial and legal decisions on behalf of a person with dementia. It is significant because dementia may impair cognitive processes over time, making it more difficult for people to handle their affairs. With a POA in place, caregivers may manage duties such as paying bills, managing investments, and making financial choices in the best interest of the person with dementia. This instrument guarantees that significant financial concerns are addressed swiftly and responsibly without judicial involvement.

Living Will

A Living Will, also known as an advance directive, is another vital document for dementia caretakers. It helps people to define their wishes for medical treatment and end-of-life care in advance. For someone with dementia, this document becomes crucial as the condition develops, and the individual may lose the capacity to convey their desires. A Living Will defines the medical care the individual wishes or does not want, such as life-sustaining therapies or palliative care alternatives. This guarantees that caregivers and healthcare personnel understand and follow the individual's desires for their medical treatment, even when they can no longer express them.

Guardianship

Guardianship is a legal relationship when a court assigns a caregiver, a guardian, to make personal and healthcare choices for an individual considered incapable of making such decisions freely due to dementia. Obtaining guardianship includes a legal procedure where proof of the person's incapacity is given to the court. Once appointed, the guardian is responsible for making choices about the person's living circumstances, medical care, and general well-being. Guardianship is a crucial obligation that offers the caregiver the legal ability to act on behalf of the person with dementia in situations that impact their daily life and health.

For dementia caregivers, these legal papers serve as protective measures that guarantee they can execute their tasks successfully while respecting the rights and preferences of the person under their care. They give clarity and legal authority in instances where the cognitive decline of dementia may otherwise generate questions and obstacles. By addressing financial, medical, and personal care requirements via these agreements, caregivers may negotiate the difficulties of dementia care with more confidence and legitimacy, assuring the well-being and dignity of their loved ones throughout the advancement of the illness.

Financial Planning

Financial planning for dementia caregivers entails vital concerns such as budgeting for care, examining insurance choices, and comprehending government aid programs. These factors are essential for managing large expenditures and delivering enough assistance for the caregiver and the person with dementia.

Budgeting for Care

Budgeting for dementia care demands rigorous preparation owing to the unpredictable nature of the illness and its long-term repercussions. Caregivers can face large expenditures connected to medical treatment, housing renovations, and professional caring services. Creating a thorough budget involves:

Assessing Current and Future expenditures: Identify current expenditures linked to drugs, medical visits, and specialized equipment. Anticipate future costs such as home care services or residential care facility fees as the condition worsens.

Exploring financing Sources: Research prospective sources, including personal savings, health insurance coverage, and long-term care insurance plans. Consider creating a separate savings account or trust devoted to dementia care expenditures.

Seeking Financial Assistance: Look into government assistance programs like Medicaid, which covers long-term care expenses for qualified persons with low income and resources. Additionally, charity organizations or local community resources that provide financial help or grants expressly for dementia caregivers should be considered.

Consulting Financial Advisors: Seek help from financial advisers specialized in elder care or estate preparation. They may give specialized assistance on managing money, improving assets, and negotiating tax consequences connected to caring expenditures.

Insurance Options

Understanding insurance alternatives is vital for lessening the financial burden connected with dementia care:

Health Insurance Coverage: Review current health insurance plans to understand coverage for dementia-related medical expenditures, including doctor visits, hospitalizations, and prescription drugs. Supplemental policies or Medicare Advantage plans may provide extra benefits.

Long-Term Care Insurance: Consider getting long-term care insurance early since plans often have waiting periods before benefits can be used. These plans may cover expenditures linked to in-home care, assisted living facilities, or nursing home care that may not be entirely covered by health insurance.

Life Insurance and Annuities: Evaluate life insurance plans with cash value that may be employed to cover care bills. Annuities may also offer a stable income stream to support ongoing caring needs.

Disability Insurance: If the caregiver cannot work due to caring obligations, disability insurance benefits might offer supplemental income to meet daily living expenditures.

Government Assistance Programs

Government aid programs provide critical help to dementia caregivers:

Medicaid: Medicaid offers health coverage and long-term care services for low-income persons, including those with dementia. Eligibility requirements vary by state and may include income and wealth limitations.

Medicare: While Medicare typically covers acute medical services, it may pay for short-term skilled nursing care after hospitalization. Medicare Advantage plans may provide extra benefits for chronic care management.

Veterans Benefits: Veterans and their spouses may qualify for VA benefits, including Aid and Attendance, which offers financial support for veterans requiring aid with everyday chores due to dementia or other disorders.

Social Security Disability payments: Caregivers who cannot work due to caring obligations may qualify for Social Security Disability Insurance (SSDI) or Supplemental Security Income (SSI) payments based on their employment history and financial need.

CHAPTER 6: SUPPORT FOR CAREGIVERS

The Role of the Caregiver

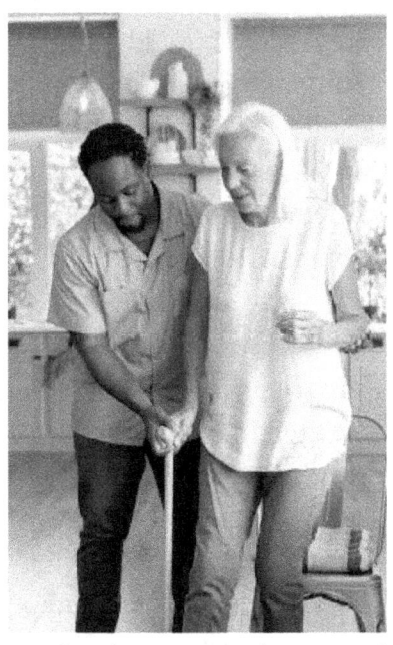

The role of the dementia caregiver is diverse and demanding, requiring compassion, patience, and specific abilities to serve those with dementia. Caregivers are crucial in giving patients physical, emotional, and cognitive care, often becoming their primary source of stability and comfort. They aid with everyday duties such as personal cleanliness, medication administration, food preparation, and changing routines as the condition develops.

Beyond physical care, dementia caregivers provide emotional support by maintaining meaningful conversation and a feeling of security for their patients. They tackle issues like mood swings, forgetfulness, and memory loss with empathy, knowing each client's particular requirements. Caregivers also function as advocates, talking with healthcare professionals, managing appointments, and ensuring treatment plans are followed.

The position needs resilience as caregivers confront stress, weariness, and emotional strain. They typically sacrifice personal time and jobs to emphasize the well-being of their loved ones. Despite these hurdles, caregivers enjoy boosting their patients' quality of life, maintaining dignity, and creating moments of joy despite the hardships of dementia. Their commitment and altruism are essential in negotiating the intricacies of dementia care, tremendously impacting the lives of patients and families.

Coping with Stress and Burnout

Caregiving for a loved one with dementia may be emotionally and physically taxing. It's normal for caregivers to suffer stress, anxiety, and even depression owing to the demanding nature of the work. Coping tactics include receiving emotional support from friends, family, or support groups geared toward dementia caregivers. These organizations give a secure area to share stories, get advice, and find comfort in knowing others understand their struggles.

Additionally, caregivers might benefit from stress management practices such as mindfulness, deep breathing exercises, or activities that offer relaxation and diversion from caring obligations. Accepting aid from others and having reasonable goals for oneself are vital in managing stress and avoiding burnout.

Finding Support Groups

Support groups for dementia caregivers provide vital emotional support and practical help. They give a forum to discuss caring problems, exchange coping skills, and learn from the experiences of others experiencing similar circumstances. Local community centers, hospitals, and online platforms commonly offer these groups, making it more straightforward for caregivers to interact with peers and access resources like educational seminars or guest speaker sessions focused on dementia care.

Respite Care Options

Respite care offers a reprieve for caregivers by enabling someone else to take over caring chores briefly. This might vary from a few hours to many days, providing caregivers time to relax, respond to personal needs, or recharge. Respite care alternatives include in-home caregivers, adult day care centers specializing in dementia care, and residential homes providing short-term stays.

Utilizing respite care minimizes caregiver burnout and promotes overall caregiving efficacy by ensuring caregivers are well-rested and psychologically refreshed to deliver the best possible care to their loved ones.

Self-care for Caregivers

Providing care for an individual with dementia may be emotionally and physically taxing, making self-care essential for caregivers to maintain their well-being and provide adequate support. Here are several crucial strategies for dementia caregivers to prioritize self-care:

Firstly, maintaining a support network is vital. Connecting with other caregivers through support groups or online forums can provide valuable emotional support and practical advice. Sharing experiences with those who understand the challenges can reduce feelings of isolation and offer new coping strategies.

Secondly, setting realistic expectations and boundaries is crucial. Caregivers often feel pressure to do everything perfectly, leading to burnout. Setting achievable goals and learning to say no when necessary helps manage stress levels and prevents overwhelming fatigue.

Third, taking breaks is not a luxury; it is an imperative. Caregivers should schedule regular breaks to recharge, whether it's a short walk, reading a book, or pursuing a hobby. Respite care services or asking family and friends for help can provide opportunities for longer breaks to rest and rejuvenate.

Fourthly, prioritizing physical health through regular exercise and a balanced diet is essential. Exercise can reduce stress, improve mood, and enhance overall well-being. A nutritious diet supports energy levels and immune function, which are crucial for managing the demands of caregiving.

Fifthly, finding moments of joy and relaxation in everyday life is essential. Engaging in enjoyable activities, such as listening to music, spending time outdoors, or practicing relaxation techniques like deep breathing or meditation, helps caregivers manage stress and maintain a positive outlook.

CHAPTER 7: RESOURCES AND SUPPORT

Professional Care Services

Professional caregivers trained in dementia care are vital in delivering assistance across diverse settings and responding to differing degrees of independence and medical requirements.

In-Home Care

Many persons choose to receive dementia care in the comfort of their own homes, surrounded by familiar environs and loved ones. In-home caregivers offer specialized support suited to the particular requirements of each client. They aid with everyday duties such as grooming, medicine reminders, food preparation, and companionship. Moreover, they establish a secure and organized atmosphere to decrease confusion and enhance involvement via activities to boost cognitive function. In-home care helps persons with dementia feel free while obtaining the essential assistance to manage their illness efficiently.

Adult Day Care

Adult daycare facilities provide a structured atmosphere during daytime hours, giving relief to family caregivers while ensuring that adults with dementia get professional supervision and interaction. These institutions have qualified personnel specializing in dementia care, delivering social activities, cognitive stimulation exercises, and nutritional meals. Participants gain from social contact and organized routines, which may increase mental ability and mood. Adult daycare services help families by offering them time for work or personal interests while ensuring their loved ones get excellent care in a safe atmosphere.

Assisted Living and Nursing Homes

For persons needing round-the-clock monitoring and specialized medical care, assisted living facilities and nursing homes offer complete dementia care services. These institutions feature personnel educated in dementia care procedures, including medication administration, specialized treatments, and aid with activities of daily living. They provide a secure atmosphere with safety elements geared to prevent straying and protect the well-being of residents. These institutions generally include social activities, therapeutic programs, and sensory stimulation to increase quality of life and sustain cognitive function.

Community Resources

Local Support Organizations

Local support groups are critical in giving aid and resources to dementia caregivers, delivering essential community-based support. One significant group is the Alzheimer's Association, which maintains chapters countrywide, including local branches such as the Alzheimer's Association of Greater Pennsylvania. These chapters offer caregivers educational programs, support groups, and respite care services, which are essential for handling the demands of caring.

Another notable local resource is the Memory and Aging Center at UCSF Health in San Francisco. This facility provides specialized medical treatment, clinical research, and support services geared to dementia patients and their caregivers. They guarantee complete assistance and access to cutting-edge research through relationships with local hospitals and community centers.

National and International Organizations

On a larger scale, national and international organizations push for policy and research funding while offering significant resources. The National Institute on Aging (NIA), part of the National Institutes of Health (NIH), sponsors research on Alzheimer's disease and associated dementias, disseminating results that influence caregiving practices internationally.

Alzheimer's Disease International (ADI) operates as a global federation of Alzheimer's organizations representing interests worldwide. It organizes activities among member organizations, including the Alzheimer's Society UK and Alzheimer Society of

Canada, to improve worldwide awareness and encourage best practices in dementia care.

Community Resources for Dementia Caregivers

These organizations empower caregivers by providing informational resources, caregiver training programs, and financial support options. Local chapters of the Alzheimer's Association offer practical seminars on controlling behaviors and accessing community resources, assisting caregivers through every stage of dementia development.

Online Resources and Tools

Online services and tools for dementia caregivers offer essential assistance and knowledge available anytime, anywhere. Caregiver Action Network (CAN) provides an online toolbox with practical suggestions, caregiver stories, and seminars addressing many areas of dementia care. AARP offers a specialized online caring resource center with articles, forums, and advice on overcoming legal, financial, and emotional obstacles.

The Alzheimer's Association's Caregiver Center provides many resources, including informative films, a 24/7 Helpline, and an online community where caregivers may interact with others experiencing similar issues. Alzheimer's Society in the UK has an online forum where caregivers may seek information, exchange stories, and discover local support services.

Technology-based solutions, such as caregiver applications like CaringBridge and Lotsa Helping Hands, enhance collaboration among caregivers, allowing them to plan chores, exchange information, and request help from friends and family. Telehealth systems provide virtual assistance via consultations with healthcare specialists, including guidance on symptom management and caregiver self-care.

These online resources empower caregivers by delivering knowledge, emotional support, and practical tools to better their caring journey, thereby increasing the quality of life for caregivers and those with dementia.

CHAPTER 8: ADVANCES IN DEMENTIA RESEARCH

This chapter analyzes the contemporary landscape of dementia research, emphasizing growing trends, recent discoveries in treatment, and prospects in dementia care, giving a complete assessment of the strides being made in this subject.

Current Research Trends

In recent years, dementia research has experienced dramatic advancements spurred by neuroscience, genetics, and technology improvements. Several important factors are driving contemporary research efforts:

Early diagnosis and Diagnosis: There is a rising focus on early diagnosis of dementia via the discovery of biomarkers and subtle cognitive impairments. Researchers are researching sophisticated imaging methods such as PET scans, MRI, and blood-based biomarkers to identify degenerative alterations in the brain before clinical symptoms manifest. Early diagnosis allows for prompt therapies, perhaps reducing disease development and improving outcomes.

Genetic and Molecular Insights: Genetic research has identified many risk genes related to numerous forms of dementia, including Alzheimer's disease. Researchers are diving into the molecular underpinnings behind these disorders to seek novel treatment targets. Advances in genomic sequencing and analytics permit large-scale investigations aiming at resolving the genetic intricacies of dementia and their implications for customized therapy.

Lifestyle Interventions: Growing evidence supports the relevance of lifestyle variables in dementia prevention and treatment. Studies are studying how food, exercise, cognitive stimulation, and social interaction impact brain health and resistance against neurodegeneration. Interventions concentrating on lifestyle adjustments and mental training programs are being examined for their potential to postpone illness onset or diminish its severity.

Brain Health and Resilience: Research efforts are increasingly focused on identifying variables that enhance brain resilience and minimize the effect of neurodegenerative processes. This involves examining neuroplasticity—the brain's capacity to rearrange and generate new neural connections—and devising techniques to boost cognitive reserve via education, mental stimulation, and social contact.

Technology and Digital Health: Combining digital health technology transforms dementia research and treatment. Wearable gadgets, smartphone apps, and virtual reality tools are being leveraged to continuously monitor cognitive performance, physical activity, and medication adherence. Artificial intelligence and big data analytics are also being harnessed to evaluate enormous volumes of data and identify trends that might inspire individualized treatment methods.

Breakthroughs in Treatment

While a definite cure for dementia remains elusive, recent years have witnessed hopeful advancements in treatment strategies:

Precision Medicine Approaches: Precision medicine strives to personalize therapies to individual genetic, molecular, and clinical characteristics. Researchers are developing tailored drugs that target particular biological pathways involved in dementia, with some medications already showing promise in clinical trials. This technique has promise for more effective and tailored therapies that might influence disease development.

Immunotherapy and Disease Modification: Immunotherapy methods, which harness the body's immune system to target and eliminate aberrant proteins such as beta-amyloid and tau, represent a frontier in dementia treatment. Monoclonal antibodies and vaccinations targeted to increase immune responses against these proteins are undergoing rigorous testing in clinical trials, presenting promise for disease-modifying therapies that might reduce or prevent neurodegeneration.

Repurposing current medications: Researchers are studying the therapeutic potential of current medications licensed for treating dementia and other illnesses. Drugs addressing inflammation, metabolic dysfunction, and cardiovascular risk factors are being repurposed based on new data connecting these variables to dementia pathogenesis. This method speeds up the timescale for medication development and enhances therapeutic alternatives accessible to patients.

Non-Pharmacological Interventions: Non-pharmacological treatments such as cognitive rehabilitation, music therapy, and sensory stimulation are recognized for boosting the quality of life for patients with dementia. These therapies preserve cognitive function, regulate behavioral symptoms, and enhance emotional well-being, combining pharmaceutical treatments to offer holistic care.

Multimodal Treatment Strategies: Combining pharmaceutical therapies with non-pharmacological therapy and lifestyle adjustments is emerging as a potential strategy for dementia care. Multimodal therapies address several components of the illness process, enhancing therapy results and improving the overall quality of life for patients and caregivers alike.

Future Directions in Dementia Care

Looking forward, the future of dementia care is impacted by continuous scientific advancements and developing healthcare paradigms:

Early Intervention and Prevention Strategies: Efforts will continue to concentrate on early detection and intervention measures to delay or prevent dementia development. Population-level programs promoting brain health from midlife onwards, along with biomarker-driven diagnostic technologies, are likely to play a significant role in early intervention efforts.

Personalized and Precision Care Approaches: Integrating customized medicine into clinical practice will become more sophisticated, with breakthroughs in biomarker identification and tailored drugs. Digital health technology will provide continuous monitoring and adaptive treatments, allowing for tailored care plans that adapt to the changing requirements of patients.

Support for Caregivers: Recognizing the critical role of caregivers in dementia care, future initiatives will focus on support services and instructional materials. Caregiver training in effective communication tactics, behavioral management approaches, and self-care practices will increase caring experiences and patient outcomes.

Worldwide Collaboration and Policy Initiatives: Addressing the worldwide effect of dementia demands coordinated efforts across international boundaries. Policymakers, healthcare professionals, academics, and community stakeholders must lobby for dementia-friendly legislation, equal access to treatment, and more significant research funding to stimulate innovation and enhance patient outcomes globally.

Ethical and Social Considerations: As new therapies and technology arise, ethical questions concerning consent, privacy, and equality in healthcare delivery will become more relevant. Ensuring that developments in dementia care retain concepts of dignity, autonomy, and respect for individuals with dementia will be crucial in influencing future healthcare practices.

CHAPTER 9: PERSONAL STORIES AND CASE STUDIES

Real-life Experiences of Those Living with Dementia

Living with dementia considerably influences people and their loved ones, changing everyday life and relationships. Real-life accounts demonstrate people's obstacles and emotional moments in managing this complicated disease. For many, the earliest phases are distinguished by minor but disturbing changes—a forgotten appointment, a missing item—that eventually escalate. These early indicators frequently spark medical visits and emotional changes as families deal with the diagnosis.

As dementia progresses, patients suffer a steady deterioration of memory and cognitive ability. Simple activities become difficult once familiar faces strangers. Yet, among these struggles, clarity, and connection may arise unexpectedly. Family reunions may elicit distant memories, briefly bridging the gap between past and present. For caretakers, each day offers both great duty and poignant moments of sensitivity as they seek to provide comfort and protect dignity.

The emotional landscape of dementia is diverse. Frustration and bewilderment may give way to flashes of elation or depression. Loss and loss pervade everyday life, both for the individual with dementia and their loved ones experiencing the slow shift. Communication frequently becomes non-verbal, depending on gestures, touch, and emotions to communicate meaning.

Navigating care options adds another element of difficulty. From in-home help to residential care facilities, choices must balance safety, quality of life, and individual preferences. Each option bears emotional weight, indicating a wish to respect autonomy while providing necessary assistance.

Caregiver Stories

Dementia caregiver stories reflect a tapestry of challenges, love, and resilience woven through the experiences of those caring for loved ones battling dementia. Each narrative unveils a profoundly personal journey marked by profound emotional and practical hurdles.

One such story centers on Sarah, who devoted herself to caring for her father, George, who was diagnosed with Alzheimer's disease. Initially a vibrant and independent man, George's decline was gradual yet relentless. Sarah navigated the complexities of managing his daily routines as he struggled with confusion and memory loss. She described the heartbreaking moments when he no longer recognized her, juxtaposed with fleeting instances of lucidity that sparked hope amidst the overwhelming responsibilities.

Another poignant account comes from Michael, whose wife, Emily, was diagnosed with vascular dementia. Their life together transformed as he assumed the role of primary caregiver. Michael recounted the adjustments, from modifying their home to ensure safety to learning to communicate effectively amidst Emily's cognitive decline. He shared the bittersweet anecdotes of their shared past, now cherished memories amidst the challenges they faced daily.

Across these stories, a common thread emerges: the resilience of caregivers. They grapple with guilt, frustration, and grief while striving to provide the best care possible. Many caregivers find solace in support groups or online communities, sharing strategies and emotional support.

These narratives emphasize the significance of compassion and understanding in dementia care. They offer light on the massive impact of the disease on the individuals diagnosed and their caregivers, who navigate a demanding journey with courage and compassion. Through their stories, caregivers like Sarah and Michael advocate for awareness and support, offering insights into the realities of dementia care and the strength found in human connection amidst adversity.

The Practical Guide to Dementia | **Juana H. Bennett**

Conclusion

In conclusion, 'The Practical Guide to Dementia' presents a thorough and compassionate approach to understanding and treating dementia. Throughout the book, the writers highlight the necessity of empathy, patience, and practical techniques for caregivers and family members. By offering comprehensive descriptions of the many forms and stages of dementia, the book provides readers with information to spot signs early and seek appropriate medical help.

One of the primary features of the book rests in its practical guidance on daily caring duties, such as communication skills, managing behavioral changes, and providing a secure atmosphere. These insights not only promote the well-being of persons with dementia but also assist caregivers in negotiating the emotional and practical problems they may confront.

Furthermore, 'The Practical Guide to Dementia' stresses the necessity of self-care for caregivers, understanding that helping someone with dementia may be emotionally exhausting. The book underlines the necessity of sustaining caregiver health and resilience by advocating for self-care techniques and seeking help from healthcare experts and support groups.

Appendices

Dementia: A general term describing a decrease in mental capacity severe enough to interfere with everyday living. It is not a single sickness but rather a range of symptoms.

Alzheimer's Disease: The most prevalent type of dementia, marked by memory loss, cognitive decline, and behavioral abnormalities.

Caregiver: Someone who offers physical, emotional, or financial assistance to a person with dementia.

Cognitive Decline: A loss in mental skills such as thinking, remembering, and reasoning.

Activities of Daily Living (ADLs): Basic self-care chores include eating, bathing, dressing, toileting, and transferring.

Behavioral and Psychological Symptoms of Dementia (BPSD): Non-cognitive symptoms such as agitation, anger, wandering, and hallucinations.

Respite Care: Temporary care offered to relieve a primary caregiver, generally via professional services or support groups.

Memory Care: Specialized care focusing on treating symptoms and providing a safe environment for those with dementia.

Advance Directive: Legal papers that define a person's desires for medical treatments and care preferences in case they cannot interact.

Care Plan: A specialized approach defining the individual requirements, preferences, and objectives of a person with dementia, as well as the caring chores and responsibilities.

Grief and Loss: Emotional reactions experienced by caregivers owing to the gradual nature of dementia and its influence on the person's skills and personality.

Support Group: A meeting of caregivers and those affected by dementia to exchange experiences, information, and emotional support.

Wandering: A frequent behavior in dementia when patients may endlessly wander owing to bewilderment or restlessness.

Validation Therapy: A strategy using empathic conversation to help persons with dementia by validating their experiences and realities.

Hospice Care: End-of-life care focuses on comfort and quality of life for persons with terminal conditions, including dementia.

Frontotemporal Dementia (FTD): A set of conditions characterized by gradual nerve cell loss in the brain's frontal and temporal lobes, impairing behavior, personality, and language ability.

Vascular Dementia: Dementia is caused by reduced blood supply to the brain, generally due to strokes or small vessel disease.

Mild Cognitive Impairment (MCI): A stage between average age-related cognitive decline and dementia, when people have notable memory or cognitive deficiencies but may still perform everyday tasks.

Neuropsychological Testing: Assessments done by psychologists to measure cognitive abilities such as memory, language, and problem-solving capabilities.

Dementia-friendly Environment: Physical environments and communities intended to help persons with dementia by decreasing confusion and boosting independence and safety.

Caregiver Help Program: Programs provide resources, education, counseling, and respite services to help caregivers handle the demands of caring.

Home Modifications: Adaptations made to the home environment to promote safety and accessibility for persons with dementia, such as adding grab bars or reducing tripping hazards.

Person-Centered Care: This approach to caring stresses recognizing and honoring the individual's preferences, needs, and values across all care areas.

Elder Law Attorney: Legal practitioners specialize in problems affecting older folks, including estate preparation, guardianship, and long-term care planning for those with dementia.

Cognitive Rehabilitation: Therapeutic methods aiming at increasing cognitive function or correcting for deficiencies in patients with dementia.

Anticipatory Grief: Emotional reaction experienced by caretakers as they prepare for the steady deterioration of their loved one with dementia.

Delirium: Acute confusion and alterations in cognition are generally induced by underlying medical disorders or drugs. They are different from dementia but may coincide.

Caregiver Burden: Physical, emotional, social, and financial obstacles caregivers encounter due to the demands of caring tasks.

Geriatrician: Medical specialists specializing in the health care of older persons, particularly diagnosing and treating dementia and associated diseases.

• Frequently Asked Questions

What is dementia?

A decline in cognitive function severe enough to impede day-to-day functioning is called dementia, a general phrase rather than a particular sickness. Memory, reasoning, orientation, understanding, computation, learning capacity, language, and judgment are all diminished. The kind of dementia that is most prevalent is Alzheimer's disease, accounting for 60-80 percent of cases.

What are the early indicators of dementia?

The early warning signs of memory loss include disorientation with time and place, difficulty planning or solving problems, difficulties finishing familiar tasks, difficulties understanding visual images and spatial relationships, new challenges with words when speaking or writing, losing things, and being unable to trace steps back, diminished or poor judgment, withdrawal from work or social activities, and changes in mood and personality.

What causes dementia?

Dementia results from damage to brain nerve cells, which may impede communication between brain cells. This injury interferes with the capacity of brain cells to interact with one another. The particular source of this injury might vary, although it frequently includes the build-up of aberrant proteins in the brain.

Is dementia preventable?

Although certain dementia risk factors, including age and genes, cannot be changed, there are lifestyle variables that may lessen the risk or postpone the development of dementia. These include frequent physical activity, a nutritious diet, avoiding smoking, keeping social contact, and participating in cognitively challenging activities.

How is dementia diagnosed?

Diagnosis typically entails a full review of medical history, physical examination, cognitive testing, and frequently brain imaging or blood tests to rule out other probable reasons. A diagnosis may entail consultations with neurologists, psychiatrists, or geriatricians.

What therapies are available for dementia?

There is presently no treatment for most varieties of dementia, including Alzheimer's disease. However, some therapies and interventions may help control symptoms, enhance quality of life, and delay the development of the illness. These may include pharmaceuticals, cognitive therapy, occupational therapy, and lifestyle adjustments.

How does dementia influence caregivers?

Caring for someone with dementia may be demanding physically, emotionally, and financially. Caregivers may endure stress, anxiety, sadness, and social isolation. Caregivers must seek assistance from healthcare experts, support groups, and respite care services to help handle caring responsibilities.

BONUS

To access this bonus, click this link below or Scan the QR Code. Please remember to leave a positive review to enhance the visibility of this book.

Thanks!

https://drive.google.com/file/d/1Z7O_iR3V4IQKOp BWd-NnJ_CEln5vtpOK/view?usp=sharing

www.ingramcontent.com/pod-product-compliance
Lightning Source LLC
Chambersburg PA
CBHW071940210526
45479CB00002B/754